Kama Sutra for Couples

Everything You Need to Know About the Ancient Art of Love Making with Beginner to Expert Techniques. Love Making and Sex Positions

Riley Ashwood

Table of Contents

Introduction

Welcome to *Kama Sutra for Beginners*. In this book, we are going to explore sex from a beginner's perspective. If you are relatively new to sex and you are looking for information, tips, and sex positions, this book will give you everything you need and more. By opening up this book, you have already taken the first step in preparing yourself for your new sex life. By informing yourself as much as you can, you will ensure you are as prepared as possible so that you will be able to experience as much pleasure as you can. At the end of the day, sex is about pleasure, and knowing how best to please yourself and your sexual partners will keep them coming back to you again and again. You are going to thank yourself for having picked up this book.

The first topic we are going to discuss is what you can expect to learn through reading this book. While you will definitely learn new sex positions for every type of sexual relationship you may find yourself in (from intimate to adventurous), you will also learn so much more than that. Having sex is about more than just the positions in which you do it, so we are going to spend ample time in this book talking about the other components of a sexual relationship. These additional components include how to decide if you are sexually compatible with someone, how best to achieve orgasm for both women and men, and how to achieve and maintain intimacy. We will also look at some extra topics that can spice up your sex life when you are ready. These include sex toys, dirty talk, and any sexual fantasies you have.

Many beginner-focused sex books will begin with complete basics- beginner sex positions like missionary or cowgirl, basic tips for reaching orgasm, and basic tips like how to have shower sex safely. I recognize that you likely already know what missionary is, how to have shower sex (from seeing it in the movies), and how to give yourself an orgasm. We are going to graze over these beginner tips but spend more time on the things that will prove most useful to you in the bedroom. I will not insult you by spending 50% of the book on explaining the missionary position in great detail, but instead, I will teach you variations and new things to try once you have mastered missionary.

Read this book with an open mind and a willingness to learn. You will gain lots of new information in these pages, and it may seem overwhelming at first. The good news is, you can always flip back to any section and read it again if you forget some of the details.

Unlocking Your Sexual Fantasies and Fetishes

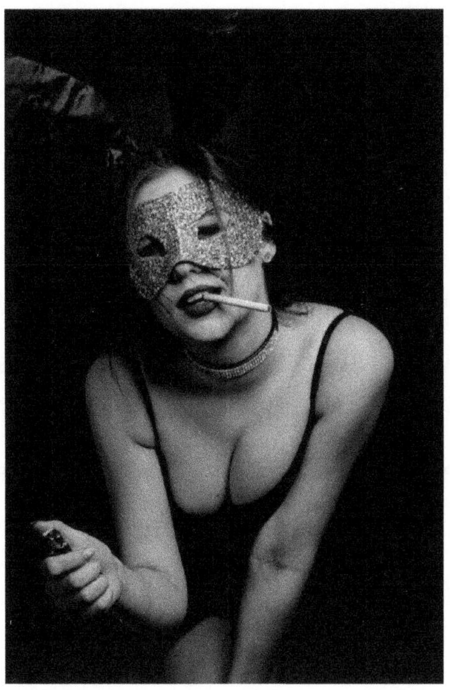

In this chapter, we will look at sexual fantasies, kinks, and fetishes. We will examine them in terms of what they are, how they can come into play in your relationship and how this can ultimately improve your intimacy levels and your sex life. First, we will begin by looking at exactly what these are.

What is a Sexual Fantasy?

A sexual fantasy is something that a person imagines or dreams of doing or taking part in. This fantasy is of a sexual nature as it usually will involve something that you would not regularly have the chance to do. For example, it could be something like having sex with a teacher as their student. In this case, this is not something that you would likely do, but you fantasize about doing it as it arouses you.

What Is a Fetish and What Is a Kink?

The lines between Kink and Fetish can blur, as the level and degree to which you enjoy something sexually can vary greatly. The things that turn people on are different for every individual and every couple, and so the definitions of kink and fetish must be somewhat flexible as well.

A kink is something that arouses you that is not considered to be the norm in your sexual culture. What is considered a kink can vary from culture to culture and between different eras in time? The terms *kink* and *BDSM* can be used somewhat interchangeably these days. Kink generally includes some type of power dynamic and dominance versus submission element. Kink is the opposite of vanilla or basic sex.

Fetishes are different than kinks in that the fetish will be more prominent to you in your arousal and pleasure. The fetish will often be more important than the person that is helping you to carry out your fetish. What this means is that a sexual fetish is a sexual attraction to an object or a body part that would not normally be associated with sexual pleasure, and this becomes a bigger focus in many cases than the partner themselves do. A fetish is required to be played out in one's sexual encounters in order for them to get off and even become aroused in some cases.

Oftentimes, you will see the terms kink and fetish used interchangeably, and this is because it all depends to what degree a person enjoys something.

How to Discover Your Sexual Fantasies and Fetishes

You are now aware of what sexual fantasies and fetishes are, but you may now be wondering if you have any personally. Everyone has sexual acts or themes that turn them on, but you must get in touch with this part of yourself in order to find out what your personal ones are. In this section, we are going to look at how you can discover your sexual fantasies and fetishes.

First, though, we will look at some specific types of sexual fantasies so that you can get an idea of what you are looking to discover. Under the umbrella of sexual fantasies is included the following, among others;

- ***Roleplay***

If your sexual fantasy or kink is role play, you likely become aroused when you imagine playing a certain role in the bedroom with your partner like a homeowner, and he is a plumber coming to fix your pipes.

- ***Domination and Submission***

If your kink or fetish is domination and submission, you likely become turned on by playing a certain role in bed-either being dominated by your partner or being dominant over them.

- ***Specific Sexual Acts***

Your kink could also be related to specific sexual acts. These can include spanking, hair pulling or Piss Play

There are so many things that can be included in these categories and so many more categories of their own. Many categories will overlap and cross over each other. For example, a police and convict role play fantasy could cross over into domination and submission play as well. By getting an idea of what is out there, you can begin to explore what you like the idea of and what you don't like sexually.

Look Inward

The first part of determining anything about yourself is to look inward and get in touch with your inner thoughts, feelings, and desires. If you are not used to looking inward and examining your feelings, it may take some practice and getting used to before you are able to determine what your fantasies, kinks or fetishes are. In order to get in touch with your feelings and thoughts, set aside some time to get quiet with your own mind.

Start to begin letting yourself fantasize about sex in general and see where this takes you. The main thing here is to let your mind go wherever it goes without trying to control it. By allowing it to drift anywhere and everywhere, you can begin to see what lies hidden in your subconscious mind.

Avoid Self-Judgement

Self-judgement can sometimes creep in when you become sexually aroused by something that is deemed unacceptable in society. When you have a sexual fantasy, it is important to remember that there need not be any shame involved- having a specific sexual fantasy does not mean that you would actually act it out in real life. Because of this, you can put your self-judgments aside and enjoy your fantasy without thinking of yourself as some sort of deviant.

Masturbation

As you are giving yourself a quiet moment to explore your mind and your desires, you may find yourself becoming sexually aroused. This is great, as it means that you have found some things that are sexually exciting to you. As this happens, you can begin to touch yourself if you wish. Masturbation is a healthy part of anybody's sex life, and there is no shame in this either.

As you begin touching yourself, allow your mind to explore your sexual fantasies, kinks, and fetishes more deeply as you become aroused. By doing this, you will be much more able to let your subconscious take over you. This is where your desires and your deeper wishes are held. Most of the time, these remain in your subconscious unbeknownst to you. It is only when you are able to access this part of your mind that you can become aware of what lies there. By doing this, you allow yourself to unlock a different level of sexual adventure and exploration. This is something that you can then share with your partner, and they can begin to know you on a much deeper level.

Research

As I stated earlier, you may not even know what sexual fantasies and fetishes are out there. By doing a little bit of research, you can figure out what is out there, what is encompassed by these terms, and what you specifically find pleasure in.

You can do research in different ways. You could explore different articles on the internet of *The Most Common Sexual Fantasies* or *Stories of the Weirdest Sexual Fetishes.* You could also look at different types of porn as there is an unlimited amount of porn available on the internet, and within this, there is a wide array of fantasies and fetishes included. The one thing to keep in mind when looking at porn is that you want to make sure you are not taking the sex you see in porn as reality. While the ideas of fantasies and fetishes can be informative to you, porn can also set unrealistic expectations for viewers related to things such as average penis size or breast size as well as how to please a woman. As long as you keep this in mind, porn can be a useful tool for exploring kinks and fetishes you never knew existed.

Even if you only find out what you are not interested in sexually, this research will still have proven to be informative.

Talk to People

Talking to your friends or people who you meet that are open about their sex lives can be another great source of information for you. The benefit to this as well is that it can give you a more realistic view of these things than you may be able to find on the internet.

You could begin by asking people about their sexual fantasies, or if they are aware of them at all. You can ask them also if they have shared these with their partners. By initiating a conversation like this, you can learn a lot about other people and their sexual fantasies or kinks.

Once you have begun to explore your sexual fantasies, kinks, and fetishes, you will be able to begin exploring them. There are many ways to try new things in the bedroom for the first time, and we will discuss this in a later section of this chapter. Exploring your fetishes is a lifelong process, as your likes and desires may change over time. Once you have found out how to be in touch with this part of yourself, you can continue to let it inform your sex life forever.

How to Discuss Your Fetishes with Your Partner

It may seem quite intimidating opening up to your partner about your kinks or fetishes or even your sexual fantasies as they are very personal to you. You may fear judgment or disgust, and you may fear that your partner will not be interested in taking part in your sexual fantasies or fetishes. In this section, I will guide you through how you can discuss these things with your partner in an open and honest way without shame or fear.

You may be self-conscious about what turns you on and

unsure of how your partner will feel about it. If you have been in this relationship for a while now and you still have not discussed these with your partner, your anxiety about bringing them up has likely only increased with time. At the beginning of a relationship, you may be hesitant to bring up things that please you that you deem unusual or not-so-vanilla. This is completely understandable, and we will discuss how to bring these topics up in conversation, regardless of how long you have been in your current relationship or marriage. The other reason could be that you have just recently discovered a new kink, and that is okay as well. If you have never acted on them before, talking to your partner about trying them can be done as a conversation about mutual exploration.

Keep in mind that many of us think our kinks are odd and embarrassing, but they are probably not as off the wall as you think they are. Fetishes may also be embarrassing to discuss, but if you are so into a certain thing that you require it in order to be pleased, your partner will surely be interested. As your partner, they are invested in your pleasure and should always be wondering how best to please you. So how do you initiate a conversation about your kinks or fetishes with your partner or spouse? The key is entering the conversation with the intention of not only explaining to them your own desires but of listening to and understanding your partner's kinks and fetishes as well.

Begin by asking your partner if there is anything that they have been interested in trying in the bedroom, or if there is anything new that they have wanted to explore sexually with you. This will initiate an open dialogue about sex and desires in general. Listen with an open mind. Your partner may be into something that you are also into! Next, they will likely ask you the same question back. Explain to them that you have wanted to try something new in your sex life with them. Explain to them what it is and how it makes you feel. Maybe you have explored this in a past relationship, and maybe that is where you first discovered this specific thing that turns you on. Maybe you have never tried it with someone else, and you would like to begin exploring it with them. If this person loves you, they care about your pleasure. Even if they may have reservations about trying something new, they are likely to be open to giving it a shot for you. Be open to exploring your kink or fetish at a beginner level if your partner has never tried it before. Sex is all about comfort and pleasure and as long as you are both feeling these two things, preferably by meeting in the middle, a good time is sure to be had by all. When explaining your kink to them, be sure to explain how it makes you feel and how it could make them feel. Explain what exactly you enjoy about it. Explain how exactly you enjoy it and what role you like to take in it. Do you like to be the dominant one? The submissive one? Allow them to ask questions and be curious. the ability to have an open conversation about sex in a relationship is essential to having a positively evolving sex life as your relationship grows and progresses. You want your sex life to grow and change along with the both of you.

We will now look at an example of this and how this conversation may go for you, in order for you to feel more secure when bringing this up. For example, say your kink is rough sex. You and your partner may have been having soft, gentle, and loving sex up until this point because you know that that is what they like, but you have learned through a past relationship that you love rough sex. You may not have tried this or brought it up in conversation before because you were afraid that your partner would have been turned off or afraid. In order to bring this up to them in conversation, you can begin by saying something like, “I used to get very turned on by having rough sex, and I would like to try it with you.”

How to Try New Fantasies and Fetishes for the First Time

When talking to your partner about your fetishes, they will likely be open-minded and willing to try it with you. This is great! In order to do this for the first time, there will be some things to keep in mind.

New Fantasy, Kink, or Fetish for Both People

If you have just discovered a new fetish or a new kink that you wish to try and you have discussed this with your partner, you can now begin to introduce this into your sex life. The positive thing about neither of you have done it before is that it can be an experience that you share with one another. By doing this, you can both evaluate as you go and decide what you like and what you dislike. For example, if you are wishing to try out a role play, you can begin by getting into the roles and using dirty talk as your characters, while ensuring that you have a safe word to use just in case someone becomes uncomfortable. A safeword is a predetermined word that you or your partner can say when one of you wishes to put the play aside and become yourselves for a time. You can use this to tell your partner that you wish to stop, to change something or to tell them something out of character. This can be used for any kink, fetish, or fantasy that you are playing out.

New Fantasy, Kink, or Fetish for Your Partner Only

If you have experience with the kink, fetish, or fantasy, but your partner does not, we will look at how to try this with your partner for the first time here.

Continuing with the example in the previous section, if you are bringing up your fetish with your partner and this fetish is rough sex, there are many ways that you can begin to introduce this into your sex life with your partner without going straight to BDSM, as they may be a little afraid in the beginning and wish to ease into it, though they are open-minded. This is completely okay. There are many degrees of roughness in sex, and it will be easy to start out by just dipping your toes in the world of rough sex to see how your partner feels about it. You can explain this to them as well. Once they are comfortable with the idea and are wanting to try it with you, you will need to take the lead. Your partner will probably not know where to start, and you will lead them through it for their first few times. To teach them as you go, try using dirty talk to make it sexier than if you just gave them a lesson in kink like a lecture at school. Begin by explaining to them whether you enjoy being in the position of masochist (pleasure from pain inflicted on you) or sadist (pleasure from inflicting pain on another person). For example, you may like having your hair pulled or having your partner dig their nails into your back when you make them feel good.

Begin by having sex as you usually would, and when it comes time that you would like it to get a little rougher, tell your partner(using dirty talk) what you want them to do. Say something like the following; “pull my hair baby” or “spank me like you're punishing me". This will make your directions sexy and fitting for the mood. Your partner may be afraid to hurt you if they do not have experience with rough sex. You can assure them before you begin that they will not be hurting you, but in fact, they will be making you feel more pleasure than usual. They will likely be excited by this possibility. This may be enough for the first time, but be sure to communicate in order to find this out. Every person is different so every person's comfort level will be different. Your partner may get into it and end up loving it just as much as you do. By beginning in this way, you can go a little further each time you have sex, and in this way, both people's comfort and enjoyment are considered.

Tantric Sex

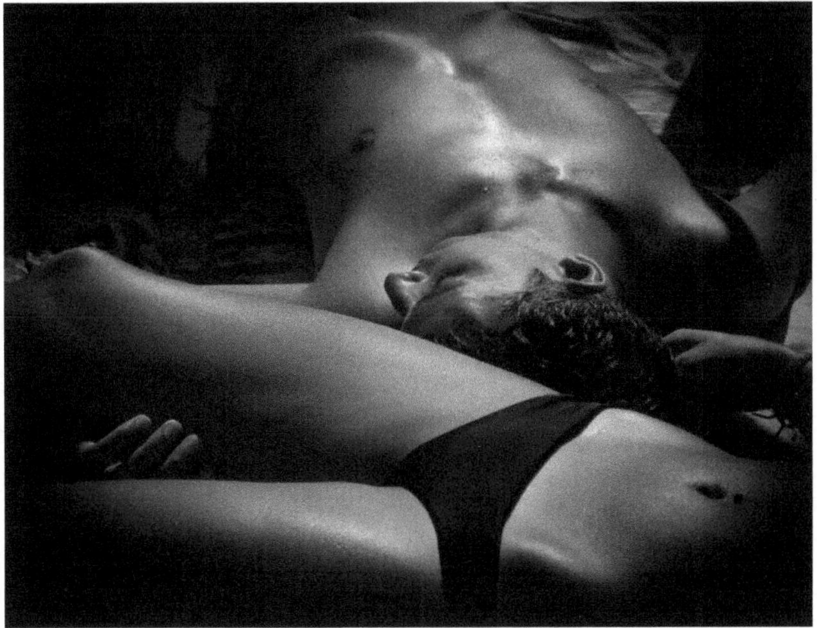

I this chapter, we are going to move on to another type of sex called Tantric sex. If you have never heard of this type of sex before, we are going to start with a little introduction.

What Is Tantric Sex?

Tantric sex is derived from something called the Tantra, which is a very old spiritual practice. For our purposes, we will be primarily looking at how the Tantra practice relates to sex and not at the other facets of this type of spirituality, though they are inextricably linked. In the way that Tantra has become related to sex, it can be viewed as a sort of new-age or *Neo-Tantra*. This is a modern take on Tantra that links it to sex and sex positions that we hear about most often today in the Western World.

Tantric Sex or Neotantra is essentially spiritual sex. It takes the old beliefs and teachings of Tantra and brings them into our modern relationships, and sex lives in order to help us better connect in our romantic relationships and to be one with our bodies and sensations. This type of sex is great for couples and long-term relationships. One of the main focuses of Tantric Sex is a mutual exchange of energy between partners. Another focus is getting in touch with the sensations and feelings of your body. It is also about removing distractions and being mindful in order to have more intense, longer-lasting, full-body orgasms. Being mindful means to bring your consciousness and awareness to the present moment. It is the state of being fully present in your body, your actions, and thoughts, and noticing them as they change. Being in this state allows you to feel the physical sensations within your body and removes the distraction of a mind full of running thoughts.

The Science Behind Tantric Sex

In Tantric Sex, everything comes down to the belief that women are generally taught to always focus on the needs of others and on taking care of others, as well as to place more importance on the pleasure of others than on themselves. It is believed that women are so disconnected from their feelings and sensations that they must begin a practice of mindfulness in order to reconnect with their feelings and sensations.

Tantric Theory states that women have a more difficult time than men when it comes to reaching orgasm. Specifically, it states that women are quite preoccupied with the duties of the household, including the children and their needs, the household and its needs, their work, their friends, and anything and anyone else in their lives. They are also preoccupied with subtle distractions such as noises or the temperature, demonstrating that they are always on high alert in an attempt to ensure everything is running smoothly and that nobody is uncomfortable in any way. This is similar to what we discussed when we looked at how to get in the right mindset for sex in terms of removing distractions and prioritizing foreplay.

In short, Tantric theory is of the belief that women are raised to focus on the pleasure and wellbeing of others and are as a result, out of touch completely with their own bodies, their own pleasure, and their own desires (these desires can be both of a sexual nature and otherwise, but here, we will focus on the sexual desires). Because of this, when it comes to sex, women tend to be unable to put aside their focus on others and turn that focus inward to themselves. When in a long-term relationship, they will be so invested in the pleasure of their partner that they will not focus on their own. Even in a casual sexual encounter, the woman will be focused on ensuring that she is giving the man a good time at the expense of her own pleasure.

To further its theories on the attention of women and their focus on many outside factors during sex, Tantric theory states that even if she wanted to, she would not have the ability to turn her focus inward. The belief is that women are unable to get in touch with the sensations of their body or their sexual desires because they have been raised to always put those aside, thus never developing the skills to do so. If she is not able to get in touch with these parts of herself, she will have great difficulty reaching orgasm. This is because she will have difficulty actually feeling what she is feeling, what she likes and doesn't like, and what she wants her partner to do in order to give her an orgasm. She will likely even have difficulty reaching orgasm when she is alone for the same reasons.

Tantric theory also has a theory concerning men and their pleasure. It is believed that men generally have short and intense orgasms and that it is possible for them to have better and longer-lasting orgasms through the practice of mindfulness as well. Tantra focuses on teaching men to be able to prolong their orgasms and make them more all-encompassing as well as to extend their pleasure overall.

Tantric sex has many techniques and methods for overcoming these challenges, and its main intention concerning women is to help them refocus their attention to themselves and their body's sensations. By refocusing on their bodies, it allows women to fully access the parts of their brain related to sexual arousal without just as equally activating the parts of their brain related to worry and concern for others.

The practice of Tantra, in general, involves being in touch with one's feelings and one's breath- almost like a meditation. Neotantra or Tantric Sex takes this idea and uses it in relation to sex. Sex with oneself or sex with a partner is done through a deep connection to oneself and one's partner. In order to do this, you practice being connected to yourself and your deeper feelings in order to feel all of the sensations in your body more easily and reach orgasm quicker and with more intensity.

Tantric sex is so useful for couples, especially those who have been together for some time. At the beginning of your relationship, you were connected by the lust, the exploration of each other, and the excitement. Now, since you know each other so well, it can be hard to reach that same feeling of discovery in the bedroom. Tantric sex can help you get there.

For men, Tantric Sex aims to help them to fully feel and enjoy their orgasms, to make them more intense and longer-lasting and to make them build up much more before releasing. It teaches women to be more present in their pleasure and as a result, their orgasms. Accomplishing these things as well as reaching a greater level of intimacy with your partner is sure to bring you to a new level of connection within your relationship, no matter how long you have been together. Devote yourselves to this practice over time (it won't happen overnight), and it will give you something to work towards as a couple and get you excited about sex with each other again.

Tantric Massage Techniques

Tantric massage is a very common way to practice tantric sex. This massage can be on one of the genital areas such as the testicles, the penis, the vulva, the nipples, and so on, or it can be done on the head or shoulders. The intention here regardless of where the massage takes place, is to focus on your breathing and get into a state of mindfulness. When you can do this, you will feel each of your partner's fingers putting gentle pressure into your skin and the sensations that this produces inside of you. By being in this state during the massage, it is a great way to get your body ready to experience sex in a deeper way, which will greatly increase the chances and intensity of orgasm.

Yoni Massage

A Yoni Massage is a vaginal massage that is intended to open up the woman to her sexuality, her pleasure, and her sexual desires. As a partner, you can perform this type of massage for your woman to unlock her repressed sexual energy and help her to get in touch with it.

This can be done in a variety of ways, but the position we are going to discuss is a Hot Water Yoni Massage. Begin by setting the ambiance, either in the bathroom with a bathtub, or around your jacuzzi. Set up some candles, some flowers, or anything that will make the surroundings relaxing and calm. Begin by having her breathe deeply and focus on her body and its sensations. You can get into the water with her for added intimacy. Begin by slowly and gently massaging around her entire vulva and her clitoral area. The key to this type of massage is to do everything very slowly. Begin to massage her clitoris slowly and not with the intention of making her come. When ready, and with lots of waterproof lube, slide one finger inside of her vagina and gently begin massaging the upper wall. Here is where her G-spot is located. Encourage her to express and release any sounds she naturally makes. Move your finger in a circular motion slowly and with your other hand, massage her pelvic area and clitoris. This connects the inner with the outer. Continue to do this and let the experience unfold with no end goal in mind. If she reaches orgasm, she can do so, but if she doesn't, she can just enjoy the pleasures that she is getting from your massage. As discussed earlier, this massage is intended to reconnect a woman with her pleasure and allow her to focus on herself and her body. After this massage, she will feel more in touch with her body, and if penetrative sex ensues, both of you will feel even more pleasure and intensity of orgasms because of how engorged and activated her vagina and clitoris will be. After doing this practice for some time either with you or on her own, she will be more in tune with her body all of the time and not just when doing this practice. This will lead to stronger orgasms overall and hotter sex for both of you.

Whatever direction this takes afterward (sex or no sex), being able to connect with your partner in this physical and energetic way will be beneficial to your sex life and your relationship as a whole. It can help the woman to reach orgasm during penetration because both of your bodies will have formed a deep connection where the pleasure is able to build both independently and together. Both of you will be in touch with your own and each other's bodies, while also being comfortable allowing your body to feel whatever it may feel and being present enough in the moment to welcome this.

Tantra is an ancient practice that has been helping couples to reconnect for decades. While you may not see yourself as someone who practices specific meditation or spiritual techniques of any sort, or if you tend to relate to more modern ideas, you may be wondering if Tantra is for you. The way that Tantra has been incorporated into sex and sexuality is actually quite a modern approach to Tantra, but nevertheless, there is a reason that its beliefs and techniques remain virtually unchanged after all this time.

Aphrodisiacs

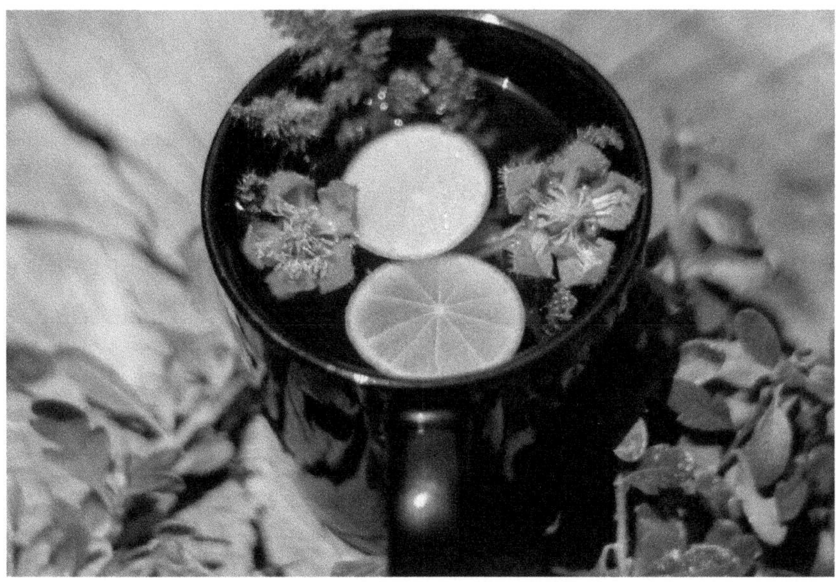

In this chapter, we are going to talk about something that can spice up your relationship and bring a new element of fun and excitement to your sex life as a couple. This new element is called an Aphrodisiac! Below, I will explain what they are and how you can incorporate them into your sex life.

What are They?

An aphrodisiac is a food or a substance that, when ingested, leads people to become sexually aroused. Many people will use these as a fun and flirty way to get them and or their partner in the mood for sex.

Aphrodisiacs work by affecting specific parts of the body, depending on which food or substance you ingest, which causes sexual arousal as a result. They can work in one of the following two ways;

1. ***Affect the Mind***

Aphrodisiacs that affect the mind work by lowering inhibitions, which leads to impulses and sexual desires. Another way that they can affect the mind is by increasing the production of certain chemicals in the brain that are associated with sex and sexual arousal or desire.

2. ***Affect the Body***

Aphrodisiacs that affect the bodywork by increasing blood flow to sexual areas of the body like the genitals or the nipples. This increase in blood flow causes feelings of sexual desire and arousal to arise for the person.

Examples of Aphrodisiacs

We will now look at some examples of aphrodisiacs so that you can get an idea of what foods and substances are included under this term.

Alcohol, Marijuana, and Drugs

To begin, we will look at two aphrodisiacs that you likely have heard of before. These are alcohol and marijuana. Marijuana and alcohol are both aphrodisiacs that work by lowering inhibitions in the mind. If you have ever been under the influence of either of these, you may have noticed that you felt more confident when it came to walking over to the bar to talk to that attractive person you had been eyeing, or that you were more forward in your sexual advances with your partner. This is because these substances lowered your inhibitions, which allowed your sexual impulses to take the driver's seat and motivated you to do things that you otherwise would not have due to the increased feelings of arousal that you were experiencing.

There are some other drugs that are known to lead to feelings of sexual arousal such as MDMA, and others that are known to actually lower libido such as some prescription drugs like antidepressants. The odd thing about alcohol as an aphrodisiac is that while it can lead to feelings of sexual arousal, it can also inhibit sexual performance, especially in males. There is a sweet spot here for increased sexual arousal before it becomes reduced performance.

Ginseng

Ginseng is an herb that is often found used in Chinese Medicine. It is often used to treat sexual dysfunction in both males and females, but it is quite strong and often reserved for males only. Ginseng can improve erectile dysfunction in men and can lead to greater levels of sexual arousal in women. It can be ingested in different ways, but the most common way in Asia is as a ginseng tea.

Pistachio

Pistachio nuts are proven to be an aphrodisiac. These nuts are found in a variety of dishes, both savory and sweet, and can be ingested whole. Pistachios have been shown to help with erectile dysfunction in men as it increases blood flow to the genitals. In women, this results in increased sexual arousal due to increased blood flow.

Other than being aphrodisiacs, pistachios boast many other health benefits, including blood pressure control, weight control, and improving heart function.

Saffron

Saffron is a spice that is used for a variety of purposes but is most often found in cooking derived from Southwest Asia. This spice is rare and quite expensive as it has to be harvested by hand and is very delicate.

At its origins, this spice has been used as a remedy for depression and mood disorders including stress reduction. Today, in men, it is an effective remedy for erectile dysfunction, and in women, it has been shown to increase sexual arousal and lubrication along with this. Saffron has been shown to be an effective aphrodisiac especially in people who are already taking antidepressants, as they often lead to reduced sexual drive and performance. If you are taking antidepressants and are experiencing a reduced sex drive, you will benefit from adding saffron into your diet if you have access to it.

Now we will move onto the fun ones, the aphrodisiacs that you have likely heard of before in the media or in conversation among friends.

Chocolate

Chocolate is an aphrodisiac that is fun to incorporate into your sex life, especially with a partner. Chocolate's aphrodisiac properties are due to the chemical compounds of cacao, which are proven to have aphrodisiac effects in women primarily.

Oysters

Oysters are a somewhat debated aphrodisiac but are

commonly referred to as an aphrodisiac in the media. This could be more due to their texture, which reminds people of other erotic things and this leads to sexual thoughts and, therefore, sexual arousal. Either way, whether it is a placebo effect or not, its effects as an aphrodisiac have been reported in some people.

Honey

Honey's mention as an aphrodisiac, dates back centuries, as it was originally used ceremonially in marriages. Since then, it has been seen as a romantic food due to its texture and its silky appearance, which elicits sensual feelings in people. This puts them in the mood for sex and love.

Horny Goat Weed

You may have heard of this one before, but its actual name is Epimedium. This comes from Chinese Medicine as well and is often used here as a treatment for sexual dysfunction in men. It has also been shown to increase sexual arousal in women. Most of the uses and studies of these substances that have been used for centuries are focused on men and their effects on men, but many of them affect women just as well.

The name Horny Goat Weed comes from its effects on goats, which is, as legend has it, how it first became discovered as goats were found to act strangely after eating this specific weed. These days it can be ingested in pill form as a libido supporting supplement.

Chili Peppers

There is a compound within hot chili peppers that is called Capsaicin (which you have likely heard of). This is what makes chili peppers spicy. When spicy food is ingested, it leads to an increase in blood flow. In this specific case, capsaicin stimulates the nerve endings of the tongue, which then leads to the production and release of chemicals in the body that are known to increase sex drive and sexual arousal. If you notice that your tongue is on fire the next time you eat spicy food, you may find shortly after that you are feeling a little more aroused than you were before dinner.

How to Benefit from Them as a Couple

Now that you know what aphrodisiacs are and what some common examples of them are, we will now talk about how you can benefit from incorporating them into your sex life as a couple. There are numerous ways to use them and benefit from them.

Trouble Reaching Orgasm

The first way to benefit from the use of aphrodisiacs is either you or your partner experiences trouble reaching orgasm. This could be due to one of you taking antidepressants, experiencing high levels of stress, or a number of other reasons. If you or your partner are having trouble reaching orgasm, ingesting an aphrodisiac before having sex may help to give you that little something extra that you need to feel maximum pleasure. By eating something spicy for dinner or by drinking ginseng tea before having sex, this will help you to get into the mood and get your body ready for sex.

Pre- or During Sex Food Play

Another way that you can benefit from the use of aphrodisiacs as a couple is to make them part of your foreplay or your during-sex fun. This will help to make it feel less like ingesting an aphrodisiac clinically as an aid for sex and more as a sexy activity that you are doing together.

For example, incorporating chocolate covered strawberries or chocolate sauce into your foreplay by dripping it sexily over your partner's body and licking it off can help you to get aroused by its aphrodisiac effects and by the sensual and heat-building act of licking it off of each other's nipples. You can do the same with honey if you prefer it. Another way to do this is by having a pistachio or chocolate-filled dessert after dinner that you can feed each other while naked in order to get each other aroused and get your bodies ready for sex.

Menu Planning

By being aware of what aphrodisiacs you can incorporate into your sex life, you can use this with your partner in order to get creative together, designing the ideal menu for your dinner one day before having sex. You can make it fun by trying to develop the most delicious menu you can while trying to include the most aphrodisiacs you can in a single meal. You can include dessert in this plan, as well. Once you have come up with the menu, you can have fun shopping for all of these aphrodisiacs and cooking your meal together before eating it and then getting into bed together. This will make you both excited for the entire process from planning to shopping to cooking to eating and then having sex! Try this in order to connect in a variety of different ways over the course of the night, and this will lead to an increase in intimacy as well as an introduction of something new and fun into your sex life.

Aphrodisiacs are often joked about in conversation among friends and on the television. They are often not taken full advantage of in the sex lives of most people. After reading this chapter, you are fully informed so that you can begin to use these things to improve your sex life. Even if you are a skeptic, you can still have fun finding new ways to incorporate these with your partner. A placebo effect is an effect nonetheless!

Sex Toys

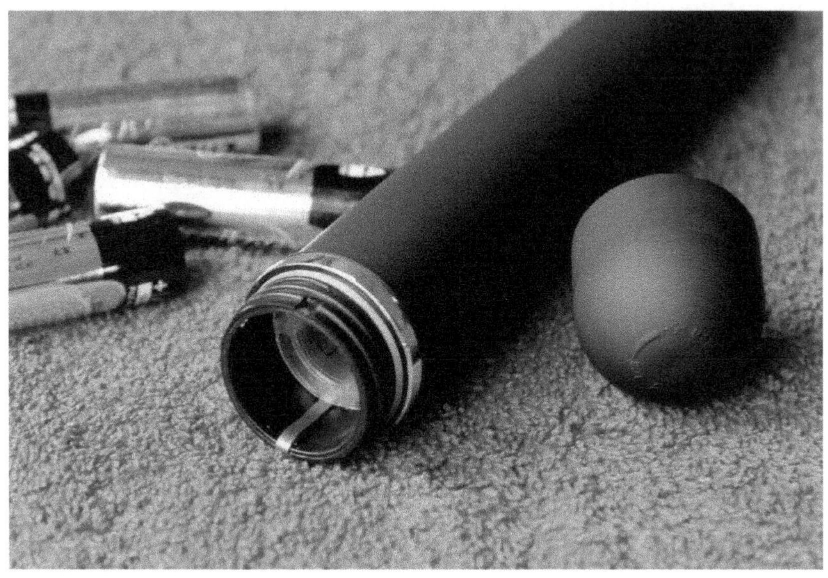

Sex toys may be something you are unfamiliar with, but they can bring fun, excitement, and new forms of pleasure to anybody's sex life. This chapter will help you to become aware of some of the sex toy options available to you and how they can be used to maximize both male and female pleasure. We will also look at how to use them safely and effectively and how to take advantage of all of their possibilities. additionally, in this chapter, we will look at everything related to sex toys and what they can offer you in your sex life with your partner as well as what you can do with them on your own. Remember, masturbation is a healthy part of anybody's sex life, even if they are in a long-term relationship. Sex toys are designed to increase and enhance pleasure; contrary to popular belief, they are not for people who need help sexually or who cannot perform on their own. The dialogue around sex toys and the fact that they are so taboo must be corrected if more people and couples want to unlock their full pleasure potential!

Sex Toys for Him

To begin, we are going to look at sex toys that men can benefit from as they are designed to be used with a penis. In this section, we are going to focus on how men can use and benefit from them on their own during masturbation, or how they can be used to please a man aside from penetration.

Cock Ring

The first sex toy we will look at is a cock ring. A cock ring was originally designed to keep a man's penis harder for a longer period of time. It does this because it is a ring made of metal that sits at the base of a man's penis, which helps to keep the blood flow inside of the penis for longer, which maintains an erection. These cock rings can be as tight or as loose as the man is comfortable with, as they come in a variety of sizes. This will also increase the man's pleasure as he will last longer.

Fleshlight

A fleshlight is another toy that is to be used by a man or anyone with a penis. This toy works by simulating a vagina or a mouth because of the way it looks and feels. Essentially it is a toy that can be disguised as a flashlight (which is how it got its name) because when it has the lid on, it looks very much like a flashlight. When you take off the lid, however, it looks like the opening of a vagina or mouth made of silicone. The man will insert his penis into the fleshlight and have penetrative sex with it as if it were a vagina or a mouth. The inside of the tube is texturized for added sensation. The soft silicone will feel similar to the skin of a woman, and this is why men find it a turn on to use this for masturbation rather than just their hand.

Sex doll

Similar to a fleshlight in some ways, is a sex doll. Instead of including only the vagina or the mouth like a fleshlight does, a sex doll is a doll that is modeled after the entire body of a woman, complete with holes in the mouth, the vagina, and sometimes the anus. It is used in a similar way as a fleshlight, where a man can insert his penis into any of these holes as if he were having sex with a woman.

The thing about a sex doll is that it is much less inconspicuous than a fleshlight or virtually any other sex toy as it is the size of a human when filled with air. It is similar to a pool toy, except that it is clearly used for sex. With this toy, it is very difficult to keep it out of sight from your partner, so keep this in mind when considering it.

Sex Toys For Her

Anything you can think of that would bring you sexual pleasure likely exists these days, and all it will take is a little bit of exploration to find out which toys you enjoy most. Don't be intimidated by all of the choices, as the purpose of all of this is to find pleasure! In this section, we are going to look at sex toys that women can benefit from as they are designed to be used with a clitoris or a vagina. In this section, we are going to focus on how women can use and benefit from these on their own during masturbation, or how they can be used to please her aside from penetration.

Vibrator

A vibrator is probably the most common sex toy available for female pleasure. Vibrators are the best choice for women who are new to sex toys and are unsure of what they may be looking for. A vibrator is a nice and easy place to start, and they can be used in a variety of ways. They are quite versatile in that they can be used by you alone, by you with a partner or by a partner to you during penetration or during foreplay.

Vibrators come in so many different shapes, sizes, and materials.

Clitoral Vibrator

There are specific vibrators for the clitoris that are called clitoral vibrators that are small and compact, portable, and easy to use. This type of vibrator is turned on with the push of a button, and then you can hold it to your clitoris for quick and intense clitoral pleasure in a way like nothing else. Having something that is designed to be used on your clitoris that is also vibrating at speeds much higher than your hands could ever reach will be quite a new sensation, but one that you won't soon forget and will be quite eager to have again.

Bunny Ears Vibrator

There is another type of vibrator that is a little larger than a clitoral vibrator, and that also has an extra protruding piece on the side of it which can be inserted into the vagina so that you can have both vaginal penetration (so that you can stimulate your G-Spot) as well as vibrating, clitoral stimulation. This type is called a bunny ears vibrator since the portion that you insert into your vagina looks a little bit like bunny ears. With this shape, you can feel both of these types of pleasure at exactly the same time! This will be a new world of pleasure for you as you may never have had both your clitoris and your G-Spot stimulated at the same time.

This type of vibrator is usually made of silicone, and the small bump-like shape that juts out the side, which is the part that touches your clitoris, is also made of silicone. The entire vibrator will vibrate when you turn it on, so you will also feel some of the vibrations on your G-Spot as well, which will give you maximum pleasure.

Vibrating Dildo

The next type of vibrator we will look at is called a vibrating dildo. A dildo is a sex toy that is designed to be penis-like in shape, and that is usually made of silicone. A dildo is used by inserting it into either the vagina or the anus. This specific type of dildo is a sort of hybrid as it has the ability to act as a vibrator as well. This is usually done by way of a small bullet-shaped vibrator that is inserted into it. This type of vibrator allows you to have penetration with vibration. Because of this, the G-Spot can be stimulated and vibrated on at the same time, which will lead to intense pleasure.

This type of vibrator is good for someone who wants a more penis-like shape without specific clitoral stimulation, as some people prefer penetration over clitoral vibration. This type of dildo can also be worn as a strap-on, but we will visit that in the next section, so stay tuned.

Dildo

We already examined one specific type of dildo in the last section, but here we will look at the dildo as a sex toy on its own, without the vibrating option. If you are not a fan of the vibration and you don't need it, or if you simply don't want that function in your dildo, a regular dildo (like we will talk about here) is an option as well.

You have the option of using a more basic dildo that is simply a penis-like object that can come in a variety of different materials such as glass, stainless steel, or silicone. These can come in a wide variety of colors and shapes- from realistic-looking penises that come in a variety of skin tones, to pink and purple banana-shaped dildos. The world of dildos is vast and contains every and any kind of penetrative device you could possibly dream of.

Dildos can be used by a woman alone while masturbating by being inserted into the vagina in order to stimulate her G-Spot. While doing this, you can also massage your clitoris with your other hand, or you can stick with the vaginal stimulation on its own. Most dildos can be taken into the bathtub or shower as well, as they are all waterproof (except the vibrating kind) so you can have shower sex with your dildo if you wish.

A dildo can be used in the vagina or the anus, whichever you prefer, and you can use the same dildo for both of these places, so you don't need to buy two. If you want to use your dildo during a solo session, you can insert it into your anus in a similar way as you would insert it into your vagina. Just be sure that when switching between the anus and the vagina, you thoroughly clean the dildo and/or your hands to prevent the chance of an infection. You could also insert the dildo into your vagina while you massage or penetrate your anus using your hand. You can really do anything you like with a dildo, any combination of sexual acts that turn you on and get you to orgasm.

Sex Toys for Him or Her

Following our discussion of sex toys for men and for women, we will now look at some toys that can be used by both men and women, either during a solo pleasure session or by a partner.

Nipple Clamps

The next sex toy we will look at are nipple clamps. Nipple clamps are usually made of silver or another metal of some sort and are clipped onto the nipples, which pinches them. The two clamps are often connected by a chain, and this causes the clamps to pull down on the nipples for added sensation.

This sex toy falls loosely into the category of sadism and masochism, which is a category within BDSM since there is a low level of pain involved in this. The level of pain can be controlled or adjusted, depending on how sensitive your nipples are and how much pain you enjoy to become turned on during sex. If you enjoy a higher level of pain, you can get nipple clamps of a heavier weight, and if you only want a little bit (especially if you have very sensitive nipples), you can get lighter ones. This depends on the type of metal they are made of, the thickness of the clamps, and the weight of the chain that connects them. If you enjoy the pinching of the clamps on your nipples because it stimulates them and makes you aroused, but you prefer not to have the chain pulling them down too aggressively, then you can opt for the light chain and clamps.

While wearing nipple clamps, you are free to touch and stimulate every other part of your own body while you experience the pleasure from the stimulation of your nipples. This is the benefit of nipple clamps as it allows for hands-off pleasure, so you are free to focus on other parts of your body.

When using these with a partner, you and your partner are both free to stimulate every part of each other's bodies, as neither of you will have to stimulate each other's or their own nipples because the clamps take care of that for you. Then, you are both free to touch each other's genitals. The only difference that may be noted between men and women when using nipple clamps is that the weight desired by men and women to achieve pleasurable pain could be different- a man may want heavier ones compared to a woman.

Anal Toys

Following our brief discussion of the possibilities of anal pleasure with a dildo in an earlier section within this chapter, we will now look at some more specific toys for anal pleasure. There are a variety of anal toys that you can use to give yourself pleasure, either actively or passively.

Butt Plug

The butt plug is a toy that is used passively to give you pleasure anally while you are busy doing other things with your hands. A butt plug is a small silicone or glass device that is inserted into the anus and is left there. This provides pleasure from the stretching of the anal opening, which, as I mentioned, is very sensitive. It also provides pleasure from the stretching of the anal canal in general, and as you move, you will feel pleasure from the pressure it puts on the inside of your anus. This type of anal toy can be used in preparation for anal sex in order to encourage the anal canal to relax, or to get a head start on pleasure during foreplay or before sex entirely. Either a woman or a man can use a butt plug during a solo session by inserting it and leaving it inserted while massaging their clitoris, using another sex toy vaginally, or (for a man) stimulating their penis. This way it can provide passive pleasure during other acts.

Anal Beads

Another anal toy that can be used for great pleasure are anal beads. Anal beads are a series of beads, arranged in order of size starting from smallest to largest, that are all attached together and that have a ring at the end, closest to the largest bead. These can be inserted into the anus all the way until just the ring is exposed at the end. What this does is allow you to insert the bigger beads last since you first inserted smaller ones, which gradually increased in size, preparing your anus for the larger sized ones. When they are inside of you, it will work similarly to a butt plug in that it will give your anus pleasurable internal pressure, as well as pleasure from the stretching of the sensitive anal opening, especially as the beads increase in size. This type of anal sex toy is an active type as it is used by being moved, providing active pleasure.

How Couples Can Use Sex Toys Together

Sex toys may be a new area of exploration for a lot of couples when in the bedroom together, even if the two people have experience with sex toys on their own. Many sex toys that can be used solo can also be used as a couple. With the advent of so many new technologies in this day and age, the potential is endless.

Using a Cock Ring as a Couple

A cock ring has another use than just for a man during masturbation. A cock ring can be used as a couple together during penetrative sex, as well. The first benefit of using a cock ring as a couple is that because it keeps a man's penis erect for much longer, the woman will be able to experience more pleasure due to a longer period during which penetration can happen. This effect will help her to orgasm from penetration because, as you now know, a woman requires a continued and prolonged stimulation of her G-Spot in order to reach orgasm.

Another benefit of using a cock ring as a couple is that there is another type of cock ring which has vibrating functions. A cock ring like this works in much the same way as the metal ones but is usually made of a softer material like silicone, and it begins vibrating with the push of a button or the flip of a switch. While the man is wearing this, it will vibrate on the base of his penis, which will be pleasurable for him and keep him erect for longer, but it will also act as a vibrator on the woman's clitoris during penetration.

Using a Dildo or Strap-On as a Couple

Dildos can be used with a partner as well as used solo by a woman, as we have seen. If a woman enjoys the feeling of being penetrated by a dildo, her partner can hold it and insert it into her vagina while she lies back and enjoys the sensation, or while she stimulates her own clitoris at the same time.

A dildo can also be used as a couple for something called Pegging. Many heterosexual couples practice Pegging, or anal sex from a woman to a man using a sex toy, usually a dildo. When a dildo is inserted into a harness that is worn by a woman around her legs and waist, it is called a strap-on. Any type of dildo can be inserted into a harness to become a strap-on. Pegging is done to stimulate a man anally when his partner is holding a dildo or wearing it as a strap-on. The pleasure potential of a man's anus is usually only discussed in relation to homosexual males, but anal pleasure is not only reserved for gay couples and should be fully explored by any man or heterosexual couple wanting to unlock the full pleasure that a man's body is capable of.

There is another kind of dildo that is used to achieve both male and female pleasure at the same time. This is a Double-Ended Dildo. This type is not worn as a strap-on but is instead used by being inserted into the man's anus while also being inserted into either the woman's anus or her vagina. Then, both people can thrust towards each other to pleasure each other at the same time. This type of dildo has the ability to please the woman in multiple ways and also has the ability to please the man to a great degree. While being penetrated in this way, the woman can also use a vibrator or another type of sex toy to stimulate her clitoris if she wishes.

Using Anal Toys as a Couple

As we previously discussed, anal toys can be used by either men or women to experience pleasure. In this section, we will look at how they can be used together as a couple.

A butt plug can be used as a couple by being left in place while having penetrative sex by either the man or woman or both. To use this as a couple, you can insert them for each other and then leave them inserted while you begin penetration. This will lead to great pleasure, especially for the woman as the pressure the butt plug places on the inside of the anal walls, in combination with the pressure that the man's penis puts on the inside of the vaginal walls come together to stimulate both the anus and the vagina at the exact same time. Also, because both of these canals have something filling them, there is an increase in the general pressure of the entire genital area, which will lead to high levels of overall pleasure for the woman. This increase in pressure of the vagina will also be felt by the penis of the man since he is inserting his penis into a smaller canal. The thrusting in and out by the man's penis while a butt plug is inserted will cause the woman and the man to feel varying levels of pressure.

A woman may be able to have a blended anal and a vaginal orgasm in this way, and if she is looking for even more pleasure, she or her partner can also massage or use a vibrator on her clitoris to stimulate all three areas at once. This will create the potential of three distinct and blended orgasms.

Sex Positions

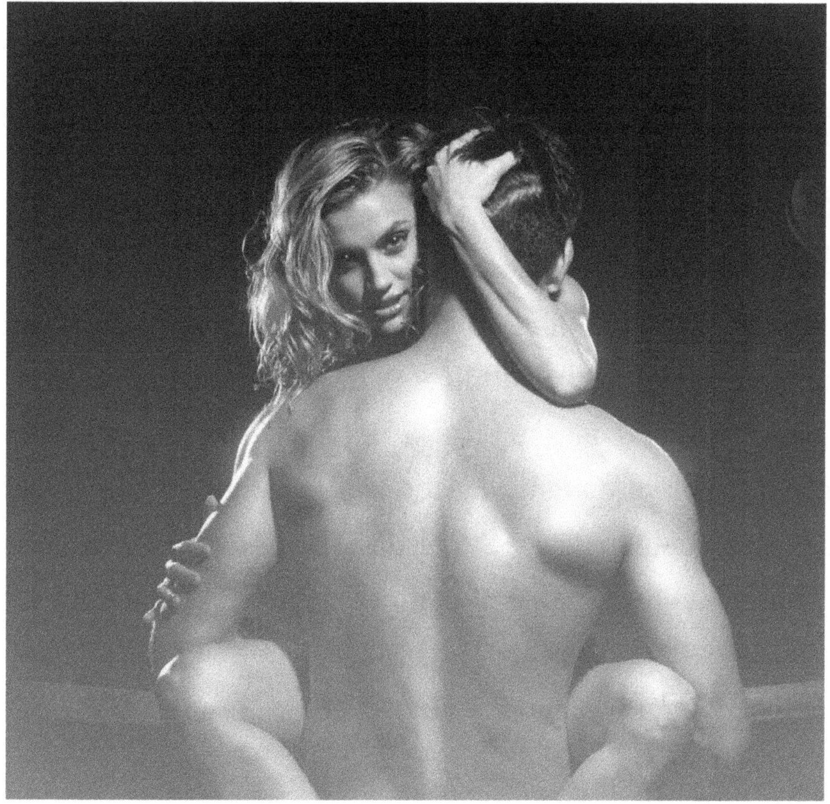

As your relationship progresses, it is important to keep sex and lust alive. When you become progressively more and more comfortable with someone, it can take away some of the mystery. This is because there is no longer the excitement of getting to know a person, and having everything you do together be brand new. Getting to this point in your relationship is fun and comforting in its own way, and is different from, but in some ways better than, the early stages.

From a sexual perspective, though, we don't want the coming of this stage of your relationship to bring with it the end of an exciting sex life. This next chapter will teach you how to maintain the lust and intimacy and keep welcoming new sexual adventures together as an established couple.

Sensual Positions for Maximum Intimacy

Intimacy is something that needs to be worked at and practiced. It is something that needs to be actively maintained and does not stay as-is when achieved once. As a couple, there are many ways to work on your intimacy, and sex is one of those ways. Sex also happens to come with many other benefits, but these positions we will explore now are chosen because they are the best for creating intimacy and connection for you and your partner.

The Lotus

Arguably the most intimate position of them all is The Lotus. The Lotus position is most intimate because of the closeness of your entire bodies, infinitely pressed against each other at all points from head to toe while being face to face.

The man sits on the bed cross-legged, his torso upright. His penis is erect and ready to get it on. The woman climbs on top of him and sits in his lap, wrapping her arms and legs around him. He holds her by wrapping his arms around her as well. With some shifting, they slide his penis inside of her. In this position, both people will be grinding more than they will be thrusting or humping. This is also what makes it so intimate. Grinding face to face while she is sitting on his lap with him inside of her, that is about as intimate as it gets.

In this position, you will not be doing any crazy thrusting, so it is ideal for a steamy make-out session, as your mouths will be so close that you can feel each other's breath the entire time. You can look into each other's eyes and whisper sweet nothings to them as you share this intimate experience.

Slow Grind

Another position that makes for a high level of intimacy and closeness is the Slow Grind position. In this position, the man sits down with his legs extended and leans back on his hands. The woman climbs on top of him, facing him and puts his penis inside of her. she extends her legs past him and leans back on her hands as well. In this position, they cannot move too much without risking his penis sliding out of her, so they are restricted to a slow grind. They both slowly grind their hips into each other and move gently. With both of their arms occupied to hold them up, they can only move their hips, and this makes for an intimate mood with no distractions of arms and legs moving about. They are seated facing each other as well, so they will look at each other in the eyes as they slowly grind and pleasure each other. You can see why this position is such an intimate one for a couple to try together.

Spicy Positions for More Adventure

If you are a long-term or married couple, you have likely tried every one of the classic sex positions together from missionary to 69. You have probably also developed a routine of your favorite positions and the order in which you do them by now. While you probably know how to please each other like it's second nature, rediscovering each other's bodies in a sexy way and learning new ways to pleasure each other is good for couples who have been together for a long time.

Reverse Cowgirl with Anal Play

This position is a new take on an old classic. Get into the reverse cowgirl position, which means that the man lies down on the bed on his back, and the woman straddles his penis; however, she is facing his feet instead of his head. From this position, the woman can grind her hips on the man's penis and control the speed and depth of penetration. To make it an advanced position; however, she will lean forward and can grab onto his ankles for support. Then, he can begin to play with her anus using his fingers or a toy. He does not need to penetrate her there; necessarily, he can just play with the outside of her anus, and she will still feel immense amounts of pleasure.

The Waterfall

The waterfall is a position that can bring something new to your bedroom routine. This position requires some flexibility and strength from both people but holds lots of pleasure potential.

The man will begin by sitting in a chair with his feet on the floor. The woman will climb onto his lap and insert his penis into her. She can wrap her legs around his waist. Then, slowly, she will lean all the way back until her head and arms are touching the floor (with pillows underneath). From here, the man will hold onto her hips and can move her body onto his penis at whatever speed and depth he wishes. He can also grab onto her breasts and massage her clitoris in this position if he wishes.

Kama Sutra: Tantric Positions for His Pleasure

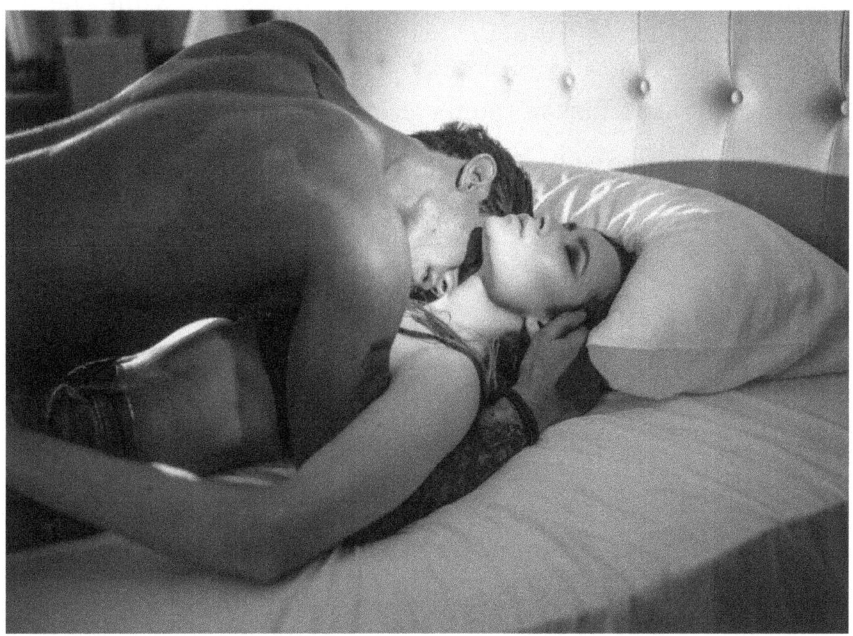

The Mare's Position

This position is a position that comes from The Kama Sutra. This position is great for the man's pleasure because of the technique it involves on the part of the woman, more than the position itself. This technique has the potential to change your sexual life forever. In this position, the man sits with his legs stretched out in front of him and his arms back, supporting his weight on the bed. The woman straddles him, facing away from him and lowers herself down onto his erect penis. Once his penis is inside of her, the woman uses her vaginal muscles to apply and release pressure on the man's penis, almost as if she is milking it. This is how it got its name. This technique makes for very pleasurable sensations on the man's penis as it creates varying pressure while he is penetrating her. It creates more stimulation on the man's penis than just classic penetration. As a bonus, this also strengthens the woman's vaginal muscles, which in time will lead to stronger orgasms for her.

Tripod Position

This position is one where the woman and man are both standing. The woman and man will both stand facing each other and the man will hold onto one of the woman's legs under her knee. The man will hold her leg raised and enter her from beneath. Because there are only three legs on the ground, this is called the Tripod Position. This position allows for maximum blood flow to the genitals, leading to great male pleasure.

Piditaka Position

This position is another Kama Sutra position, that requires some flexibility but is relaxing once you get into it. The woman lies back on the bed and lifts her knees, putting them on the man's chest. The man will get on top of the woman and holds her knees against his chest. The man will put his knees on either side of her buttocks and enter her from this position. This position is good for male pleasure as the vagina is narrowed while the woman's legs are up, which feels great on his penis.

Hanging position

This position is similar to the standing position, but it is different in that it involves a little more support. The man will stand up with his back against a wall, with the woman standing and facing him. The woman will jump into the man's arms and he will hold her up by her buttocks. The woman will extend her legs behind her and rest them on the wall. This position feels great for the man since the woman's vagina is closed up and this makes a tighter environment for the penis.

The Bent Position

The woman will lie down on the floor and lift her legs up, bringing her knees to her chest and widening them. She will hold onto her legs under her knees to keep them lifted. The man will crouch low in a squat position and lean forward to enter the woman from below. He can hold onto her legs for support as he thrusts into her. Since the woman's legs are lifted, this position feels great on the man's penis.

The Cow Position

The Cow Position is a position where the man will enter the

woman from behind. The woman will lie face down on a bed with a pillow underneath her hips to lift her buttocks off the bed a bit. The man will get on top of the woman and enter her. This position is good for male pleasure since it provides him with the opportunity to control the pace and the depth.

Fixing A Nail

The woman will lie on her back and the man comes over top of her and lifts one of her legs. He will lift her leg so that her foot is planted on his forehead. He can then enter her from the front while keeping her foot on his head. As he thrusts into her, she will alternate her feet on his head and this will change the feelings for each of them, providing them with variety.

The Peg

The man lies on his side and the woman lies facing him on her side, with her head towards his feet. The woman will lift her knees towards her chest and place one of her legs underneath the man's legs and have the other on top of his legs. Essentially, she is hugging his legs with her entire body. She slides up so that her vulva is next to his penis.

When aligned properly he can penetrate her and can achieve depth and control as she is positioned perfectly for his penis to enter her. The woman wraps her arms around his legs and he can use his hands and arms to help with his thrusting.

Kama Sutra: Tantric Positions for Her Pleasure

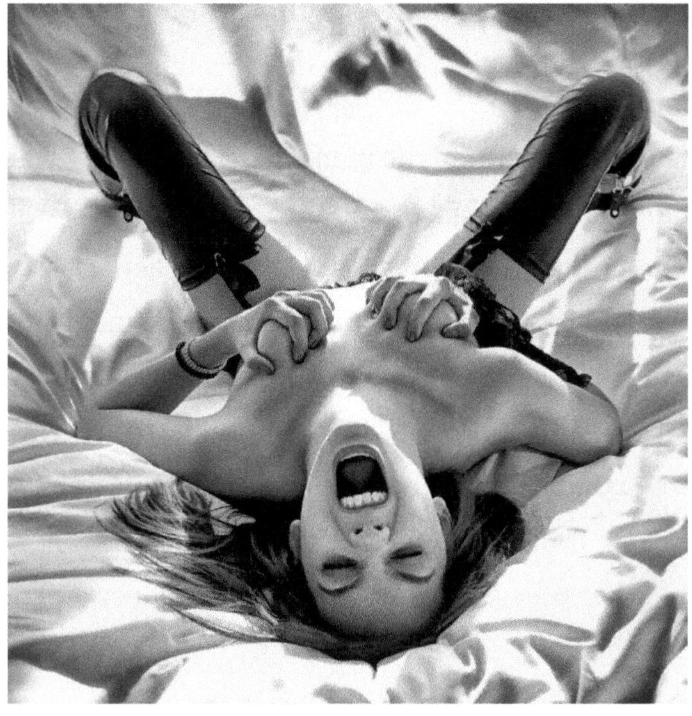

These positions that follow are best for the female orgasm and the pleasure of the woman. For great pleasure for the woman, positions that maximize G-Spot contact, as well as positions that allow for simultaneous clitoral stimulation, are best.

Standing Suspended

This first position is a position that comes from the Kama Sutra. This position is great for the female orgasm because of the angle that the man's penis enters her vagina and also because the man is in control in this position so the woman can relax and enjoy the pleasure he is bringing to her body.

To get into this position, the man will stand facing a wall with the woman standing in front of him, her back to the wall. She will then jump into his arms and wrap both her arms and her legs around him. Once here, he can insert his penis into her vagina while holding onto her buttocks or underneath her knees. He can lean her back on the wall in front of him for support so that he does not have to support her entire weight in his arms. If he holds onto her underneath her knees, this will open her up so that her vagina is easily accessible. The fact that she is suspended coupled with this will make it so that there is deep penetration occurring, and this will be pleasurable for both the man and the woman. Deep penetration is great for the female orgasm because there are two places located deep within the vagina that, when stimulated, lead to a very intense orgasm for her. The penis must achieve continuous deep penetration in order for this to happen and in this position, it is quite possible.

The Peasant

This position is great for the woman as she will receive clitoral stimulation as well as penetration. To get into this position, the man will sit on the floor or the bed and the woman will sit on top of his lap. The woman will spread her legs wide and the man will insert his penis into her from behind. The man will reach around her and stimulate her clitoris while the woman grinds on his lap.

The Rider Position

The man will lie on his back and lift his knees to his chest, spreading them wide. The woman will then sit on the man, underneath his bent legs and sit on his penis. She can hold on his bent knees for support, and grind on his penis or lift her body up and down on him. This position is great for female pleasure since she can touch her clitoris or the man can stimulate it for her. It is also pleasurable for her as she can control the movement.

Indrani

This position is more acrobatic than many other Kama Sutra positions. The woman will lie on her back and the man will kneel in front of her, near her legs. The man will lift her up by the buttocks and put his penis into her. He will hold onto her thighs to keep her buttocks lifted off of the bed. This position leads to interruptions an changes in blood flow, which will make the woman feel immense pleasure.

Milk And Water Embrace

This position is sensual and romantic, while also allowing for clitoral stimulation. The man will sit in a chair and the woman will sit on his lap, facing away from him. The woman and man will both grind their hips into each other and the man can reach his hand around and stimulate her clitoris.

The Yawning Position

The woman lies on her back and spreads her legs out as wide as she can. The man will enter the woman from the front with his knees underneath her hips. He can lean forward and their faces can come close together int his position.

The Rocking Horse

This position is a woman on top position. This makes it easier for her to feel pleasure since the angle of the man's penis inside of her will hit her G-Spot. The man sits down on the floor with his arms outstretched behind him. The woman will straddle the man, facing him. She will hug his thighs with hers and move her hips to control the thrusting. Since they are both sitting up, this position makes for a tight embrace.

The Cross

The woman lies on her back with one leg extended straight

into the air. The man kneels in front of her, straddling her leg that is extended on the bed and holds onto her other leg which is in the air. He can then move his body forward between her two legs until he is close enough to insert his penis into her vagina. He can hold her legs spread with his body, straddling one of them and placing the other one on his shoulder. By doing this, his hands will be free so that he can play with her clitoris, massage her breasts, rubbing his hands up and down her body or whatever they please.

The Yab-Yum Position

To continue our exploration of Tantric Sex, this next position is a very versatile and introductory position that beginners and masters alike use daily in their practices. This staple position of Tantric Sex is called the Yab-Yum position. You can do this position with clothes on or without. You can use it in a non-sexual moment of connection with your partner, you can use it get into the mood for sex, or you can use it as a position during sexual intercourse itself.

You can do this position anywhere, whether on a bed or on the floor, whatever is most comfortable. First, one partner sits cross-legged, and then the other partner sits in their lap, facing them, with their legs wrapped around their partner's waist. From this face to face position you can see deep into your partner's eyes, you can feel their breath as their chest rises and falls, and you can feel and sense all of the small movements and sensations of their body that you would not otherwise perceive. Get quiet in this position together to start. Just sit and experience this closeness, take in everything with each other and let the moment evolve; however, it does. Let it lead to whatever it leads to. Maybe beginning this position fully clothed and with the intention of just connecting spiritually will lead to such an intense moment of connection that you will rip each other's clothes off and have the best orgasms you have ever had because of this connection. Maybe you stay in this position with clothes on, and you feel closer emotionally. Either one is perfect. If you want to do this position solely for the purpose of penetration, try beginning by syncing your breathing together before starting to get really into the humping and the coming. This will make the position somewhat Tantric, at least, and will lead to more satisfying orgasms. When getting into this position for the purpose of sex only, begin already naked with your partner and get into the position as explained above, but make sure to have the man on the bottom and the woman on top. The woman, as the top, will need to adjust her hips in order to align your genitals with hers to allow for penetration. Once the penis is inside of the vagina, you will be linked in this tight, extremely close position. Now you can begin to thrust and grind and grope and everything else that pushes you both over the edge.

How to Last Longer

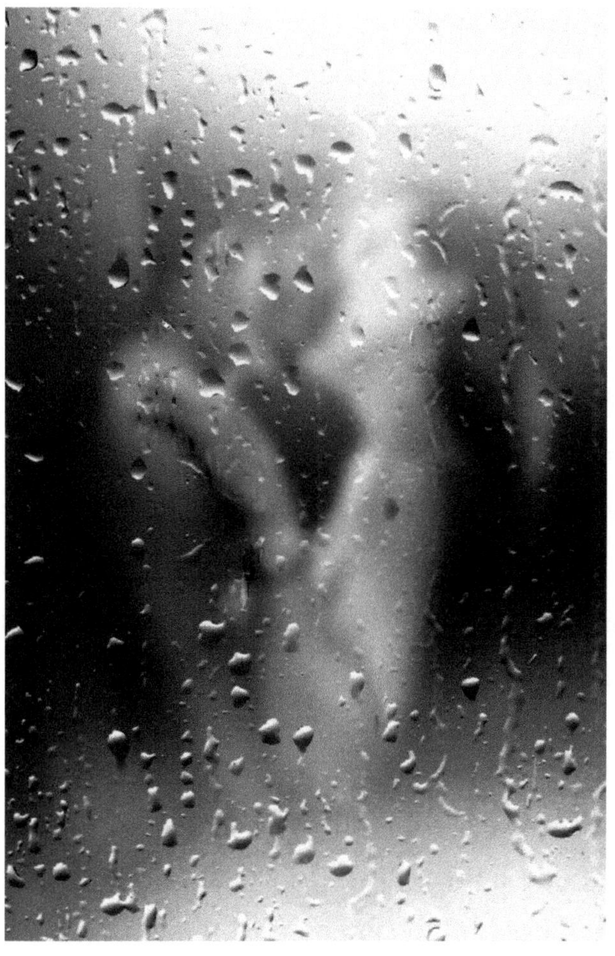

There are many theories regarding how to last longer and how to stay harder, and we will look at a few of the most effective ones now in this section. In order for both men and women to get the most out of sex and the most enjoyable orgasms, it comes down to the man's ability to last during sex.

If the time it takes a man to orgasm is quite short, then the pair will have to wait until his refractory period is over before he will be able to have an erection again. During this time, the woman will still be able to be aroused and have an orgasm, but penetrative sex will not be possible. Thus, in order to have the most pleasurable and (and also more intense) orgasms and sexual encounters, I will now present some tips and tricks that the man can use to last longer in bed.

Edging

Edging is a technique that a man can use to hold off an orgasm to make himself last longer and therefore keep his erection for longer. In order to do this, he must be aware of his body and be in touch with the different feelings it has. This is similar to what we discussed earlier when talking about mindfulness and how it relates to sex.

When the man reaches a point where he is getting very close to orgasm, he will stop, or the woman will stop whatever they are doing, and he will have to take a deep breath, compose himself and hold off his orgasm. Holding back will give him time to cool down a little and come back from the edge of orgasm. During this time, while he is cooling off, he can continue to touch the woman, or the woman can touch him in other places, as long as it doesn't make him orgasm. When he is ready and has successfully held off his orgasm, they can then continue with whatever sexual acts they were doing before. Then, when he reaches the point where he is about to orgasm again, he will have to hold off once again. This can continue as many times as he can until finally one time, he will let himself reach orgasm, and it will be much stronger and much more intense than if he had just let himself reach orgasm the first time.

This may be difficult to accomplish the first number of times because it can be hard to hold off an orgasm when you are very close. It will take practice to be able to do this technique, and especially to be able to do it multiple times over in one session. The man will have to communicate with his partner so that she knows not to keep stimulating him to the point of orgasm, especially if she was giving him oral or something of the sort.

Going to the Gym

Another way that a man can increase his endurance sexually is by going to the gym. Physical fitness is strongly related to sexual performance and endurance, so getting to the gym at least a few times a week will help him to last longer in bed, keep his erection longer and even to be able to thrust for longer because of the cardiovascular aspect that penetrative sex comes with. This will be beneficial for both of you.

Beyond the Bedroom

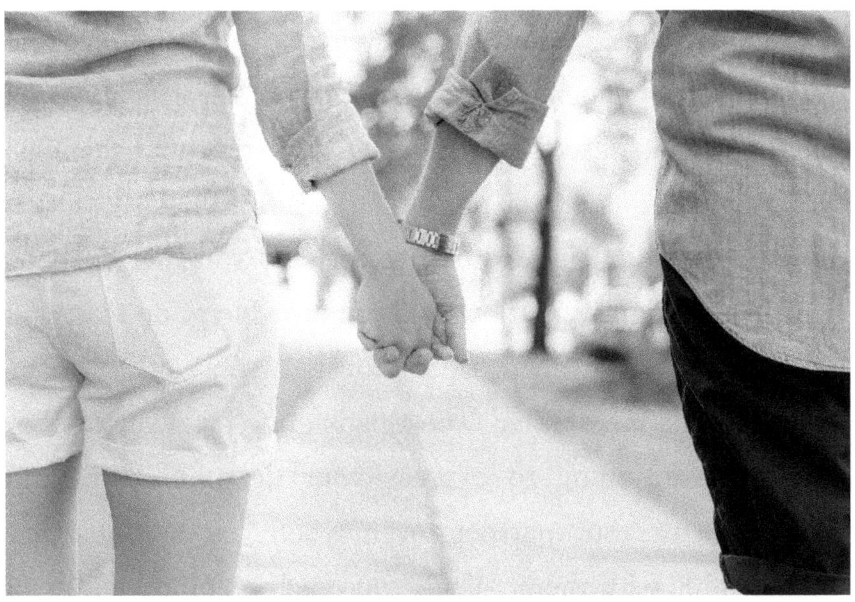

As a long-term couple, it is important that you remain intimate with each other not only in the bedroom, but outside of it as well. Since a relationship is about much more than the sex, your emotional intimacy is a large part of what keeps you together. As we discussed at the beginning of this book, there are different forms of intimacy. Until now, we have focused on physical or sexual intimacy, but now we are going to switch over and focus on the other types.

Emotional Intimacy

Just to remind you, emotional intimacy is the ability to express oneself in a mature and open manner, leading to a deep emotional connection between people. This type of intimacy is about being able to express yourself verbally using language that describes your deep thoughts and feelings. When you are able to express yourself to your partner, you create a sense of understanding between you that deepens your connection. When both of you are able to do this, you will maintain that deep connection between you. Intimacy must also be maintained, and this is done by ensuring that you are continuing to express your deep thoughts and feelings with your partner, even when you become very comfortable with them. When you reach a point where you feel like you know each other so well that you can read each other like a book, it is still important to be open verbally with your partner to keep the lines of communication open.

Expressing yourself verbally can be done by saying things like "I love you" or "thank you for being there for me." When you do this, you are reminding your partner how you feel and that you appreciate them. This is important to say, even if you know that they know how you feel. It is still nice for them to hear it from you. This creates deeper emotional intimacy. This can also be done by expressing yourself in terms of other things like why you had a bad day, what you are nervous about or what you want to share with them. Having a person close to you of this sort allows you to have someone to express yourself to, and they can express themselves to you. By doing this, you not only are able to express yourself in a healthy way, but you also are maintaining the relationship in a deep way.

Intimacy Beyond The Bedroom

There are some ways that you can maintain a good level of emotional intimacy with your partner, in order to ensure that you remain connected and in love for as long as possible. Below, I have outlined some of these ways.

Spend Time

The first way is to spend time with your partner doing things that both of you find enjoyable that you can share. When you spend quality time together, even if you are not doing anything extremely exciting, having time to simply talk and connect will help you to maintain your connection with each other and continue to know each other on and keep level as you both change and grow.

Be Curious

This brings us to our next point, which is to stay curious. Remaining curious in your relationship is one of the most important things you can do. By remaining curious about your partner and making an effort to get to know them over and over again, you will keep your relationship interesting, and you will keep knowing your partner even as they may change. This goes for every part of them, from their likes and dislikes about food, in bed, with television shows and so on.

You also want to remain curious about your relationship. By remaining curious about your relationship, you can consistently ensure that you will be giving your all and making it the best relationship it can be. Remain curious about what you can do better and what is working well in your relationship with your partner.

As you continue on in your relationship with your partner, you never know when the knowledge this book has bestowed on, you will prove useful. You may want to try something new on an anniversary getaway and think of the perfect position to try (from chapter 9 or 10), you may be having a discussion with your friends about marriage and sex and you may think of how you learned that intimacy must be maintained and worked at (chapter 1) in order to remain strong. This knowledge will remain in the back of your mind until the time when you need it most, and then it will pop to the front of your mind in order to help yourself, your partner, or your friends.

You can never be too knowledgeable about sex and

relationships, and by taking the step to read this book in its entirety, you are only helping yourself out for the rest of your life- your sex life, your romantic life, and your life in general.

How To Introduce Couple Games Into Your Bedroom

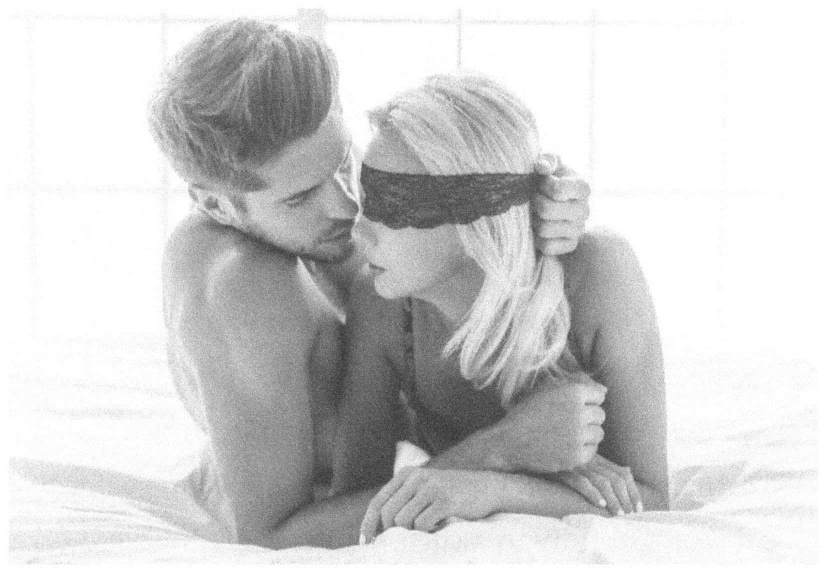

Long-term relationships and residing in the same house bring loads of everyday habits into our lives, difficulties start to extinguish passion, and soon enough sex has the risk of becoming that same “Saturday habit”. This happens frequently because daily matters and life complications dwell so much in our thoughts than romantic evenings together, as happens in the first few months of a candy-bouquet relationship period.

Unspoken discontent, unresolved problems or accumulated

aggression - all this must not be in your family life, because they are followed by quarrels, resentment, a cold and insipid bed. Sexual games are a way to get rid of daily stress, get pleasure, support the sensuality and sexuality, and at the same time not offend each other, but rather ignite. Role-playing games in bed make it possible to transform into a character and act as you would never dare in everyday life. This transformation makes it possible not to be shy, not to select words and actions, because you both understand that this is only a game.

Role-playing in bed can solve some family problems. How does it work? Roles for the game can be very different, the plot is much more important. For example, in each couple, one partner always dominates. In the role-playing game, you have the opportunity to switch places: if the husband takes decisions in everyday life, then become a strict teacher and punish him for his bad behavior. Also, a common problem in relationships, when we release the anger and discontent accumulated over the day on a partner, although a loved one is not to blame for your failures at work or other individual areas of life. So that problems outside the home do not be reflected in the relationship, transfer them to the game. If a man comes home after a heated debate with his boss, let him be the boss that night and to write you a few reprimands.

Preparing For A Role-Playing Game: Script, Rules And Inventory

First of all, think about the difficulties and innuendos in your life with your partner.

If you have never played erotic games before, this approach will help you pick up the first roles and relieve tension in the plane of relations where it has accumulated. Incorrect roles or scripts can ruin everything. Imagine a man is constantly depressed due to the fact that his girlfriend has been you swear at him with the reason and without, and here he is offered to play mistress and her page-boy - the same situation that usually. Even if a man agrees, this game is unlikely to bring him pleasure, which, as in any sexual intercourse, should be mutual.

Try to carefully lead your partner to what worries him, to identify painful points, catch random phrases, but you should not talk about it openly, because you risk turning everything into a small home scandal, rather than a fun game. Next, select the roles that would enable you or your partner to "recoup." It will not be superfluous to learn about his fantasies, but absolutely everyone has them. So that the game does not come to a standstill or go in the wrong direction (for example, you should have been mistress, and then the man took the initiative again), write a simple, uncomplicated scenario. It is not necessary to think through all the dialogues to the smallest detail, but the general direction should be determined.

Sexy Outfits Play An Important Role In Erotic Games.

Another option to decide on the roles is to delve into yourself: think about what you would like to try, what erotic fantasies visit you, what kind of dress or atmosphere you like most.

The next stage is - outfits. Dressing up is a lot of fun. And understanding what kind of clothes can arouse your sexual desire can make this activity even more fun and enjoyable. Even the most ordinary objects can be filled with sexual vibration. Everything is simple here - either rummage through your own closet in search of suitable clothes (for example, you will definitely find something for the role of a teacher or boss) or look into a sex shop (not every house has a nurse's robe or a pilot's uniform). When you have figured out the costumes, think about what equipment may be needed so as not to run around the apartment in the middle of the game in search of a pointer, stethoscope or pipi aster - everything should be at hand

Mandatory Role-Playing Rules

- The game begins a few hours before the action. Send a thematic message to your partner (for example, "Doctor, I have a headache, can I make an appointment with you tonight?") - at this moment you are already playing, so exclude the everyday messages "Buy bread". Similarly, you can throw a secret note to your partner, but you need to make sure that he will find it. It will be a shame if you put it in your trouser pocket, and he put on jeans.
- Do not start if you are not sure that you will reach the end. The worst thing is to tease each other with messages during the day and change your mind at the last moment. Such turns will not benefit your relationship.
- Do not change clothes and do not get ready in front of each other. You should meet for the first time already in full uniform and outfits, otherwise, the "magic" will not work.
- Play to the end. None of the partners in the middle of the game can take off the suit and get out of the role. Firstly, sex runs the risk of passing as usual, and not playing the psychological role for which, everything was started. Secondly, you can offend the efforts of a partner, which will only aggravate problems in the

relationship.

- Improvise. If you initially did not have a ready-made script, or it was not implemented, and the game slows down, do not freak out. The phrases "I don't know what's next," "Think of it yourself," "Maybe you can play along with me?" – they are a taboo! It's better to think in advance where the plot might go, and what to do in such cases. In any case, even if you found the problem of interpersonal communications during the game, do not concentrate on it, urgently turn your attention to any aspects that pleasantly excite you in this situation, move the focus to the exciting details, to immerse yourself in the game deeper and not lose your sexual mood. You can reflect and gently discuss all points for improvement afterward, in a more suitable atmosphere.
- Do not try to be a great actor. To read the monologues from Hamlet in front of the partner is completely unnecessary. Focus on the main goal of the game - quality sex. If you are playing not as George Clooney, believe me, the partner is unlikely to notice this and certainly will not criticize you.
- Do not go over the role of others. If the partner dominates in the scenario, do not drag the blanket over yourself. Similarly, if you dominate, - do not let the partner go over you, you will have to be tougher,

but do not go too far - for inexperienced players, the line is rather thin. It's best to clarify the rules in advance.

- Do not undress ahead of time. If you threw off clothes from each other at the very beginning, the game already failed, because the very interesting stage of flirting was lost.
- It may sound corny, but some erotic games, especially with the use of BDSM toys, require to have "stop" words. The word should be simple, but atypical for the script. If you play, for example, in a clinic, then you should not choose a “dropper” with a stop word, it's better to choose something out of the ordinary, for example, a “bullfighter” - it's unlikely that you were going to discuss the bullfight in the script.
- It is preferably that you will be home alone at this time; the phones should be shut down.
- You should be as tactful as possible, sometimes even an innocent joke can bring down the whole mood, and then the partner in the future will completely refuse such entertainments.
- Don't think about anything extraneous, if at the height of the game a kitty instead of “murmur” suddenly says that tomorrow she needs to call on her mother, then this greatly disturbs the mood.

Roleplaying Sex Games

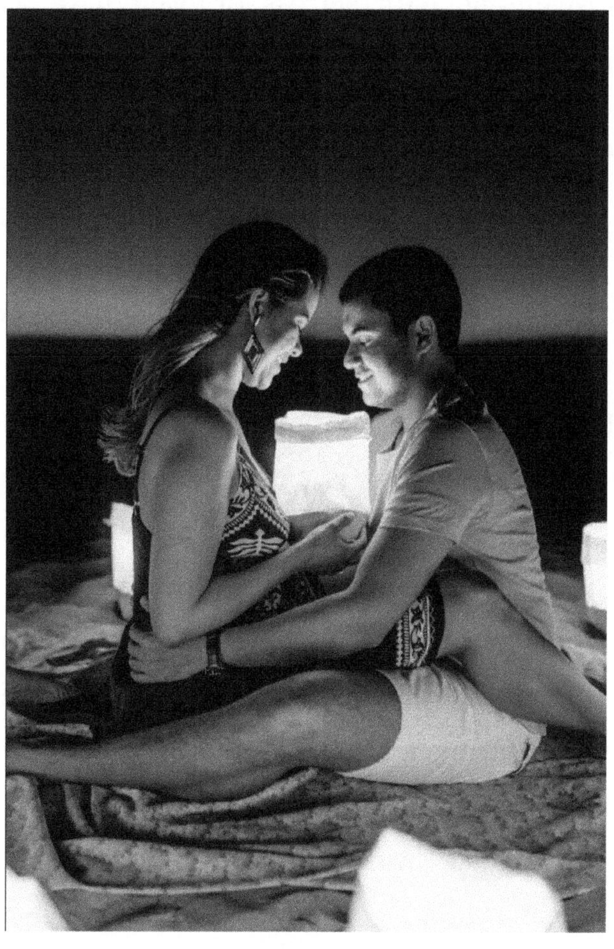

One of the easiest and fun ways to overcome sexual inhibitions is role-playing. Sexual role play is a game that involves acting out sexual fantasies using different roles that may be completely unlike the individuals in real life. The intensity of the play depends on the participants. You can choose to role-play using makeshift props or go into elaborate preparations complete with scripts and matching costumes for each character in the play. However, you don't need to be an award-winning actor/actress or even have any prior experience in acting to enjoy sexual role play.

The Process

Bring Up Your Mutual Sexual Fantasies

Unless you want to take your partner by surprise and hope that they play along, it is usually better to brainstorm different ideas and scenarios with your partner. Come up with what you each think is agreeable. We all have sexual fantasies even if we don't actually want them to happen in reality. But these fantasies could be your guide to enjoying role-play with your partner. Perhaps you wish your masseur or masseuse would be a bit more daring and take things just a bit farther during your massage sessions, or you have always had an eye for one of your teachers back in college. Share those fantasies with your partner and see which ones both of you can act out.

It is crucial to do this because one partner's idea of role-playing may be too strong or kinky for the other. But when you talk things out together, you will figure out what works for both of you. Anyway, it is a good idea to remain having an open mind and think of it all as mere fantasy and nothing more.

You can start with simple settings at first. Getting into too many details and imagination may be too daunting for you or your partner and defeat the goal of sexual role play. Start with something that can be done in a familiar setting such as your home or a nearby restaurant or bar. Select simple roles/characters and scenarios such as:

- A lonely businessman and the comforting sexy woman at a bar or restaurant.
- A pervert teacher and the naughty student in a class or the teacher's office.
- A nurse and her sick patient in a hospital bed.
- A house owner and his sexy maid in the living room or kitchen.

Dress the Part If You Wish

Go ahead and dress the part if it will help you to play the part more realistically. You can buy hats, wigs, and other costumes from costume shops, online, or adult shops. While costumes can add more excitement and fun to the whole idea of role-playing, they are not a requirement. Only get them if you think you really need them. Moreover, you may not have extra money to spend on costumes and props or you just want to keep things simple. Several roles require little to no costumes (a stranger at the bar, being on a blind date, and so on).

Make It Kinky If You Wish

Some sexual role-plays (such as officer and criminal, teacher and student, boss and secretary) are more about power and dominance. One partner (the dominant) gets to have their way with the other (the submissive). If you want to explore sexual dominance or kinkiness in a more relaxed and playful atmosphere assume the dominant/submissive roles using any character of your choice.

However, role-play is not all about power exchange. You can choose to skip any role that tends to portray the dominant/submissive attributes.

Start Slow

As always, it is best to start anything new with baby steps. It may feel too unreal, ridiculous, or just plain silly to get all dressed up and act like someone else. But you don't have to dress up to start with. Playing pretend may seem like a childish thing to do, but if you let go and play along for just a little while, you may discover that you are actually turned on by the idea of picking up a stranger at a bar, for example (even if you've known this "stranger" all your life).

Even if you totally buy the idea of sexual role play, it is wise to start slowly. You can begin by sending a raunchy text or sext detailing your sexual fantasy to your partner. This can be another form of foreplay. If you are a shy person, you can use this medium to open up communication on potentially awkward or embarrassing sexual subjects.

Let Your Character Use Dirty Words

There is no movie director here; it's just you and your partner. That is why you don't need to be uncomfortable if you get your first few lines completely wrong. Feel free to laugh about it if you fumble or make mistakes. No one is taking a score. Just let yourself ease into character and the words will flow naturally. You may or may not know how the fantasy will end. In any case, simply let your imagination guide you into what your character will say and say them without reservation. Even if you don't like profanity or filthy words, your character may like them. Permit your character to say what they need to say to make the game fun and exciting.

Sexual Roleplay Ideas

Here are a few sexual roleplay ideas to help stimulate your imagination and get the ball rolling. You are welcome to tweak them to suit you and create your own dirty dialogues along with it. You can use the dirty phrases in parenthesis as part of your sex dialogue.

1. Play the role of a firefighter who just rescued your partner and is rewarded with sex. (Dirty phrase: “You saved my life. The least I can do is to offer you my dick/pussy.”)

2. Play the role of a cop. Your partner is trying to get wriggle their way out of a speeding ticket. (Dirty phrase: “The only way to get out of this is to please me.”)

3. Play the role of a prostitute who’s just having sex for the cash. (Dirty phrase: “Show me the cash and I’ll give you good pussy/cock.”)

4. Pretend you came for a sleepover at your friend’s and snuck out to have sex with your friend’s sibling. (Dirty phrase: “Shhh... come have a taste of this cock/pussy before someone sees us.”)

5. Pretend that you are a client getting a massage from your partner who is a masseur or masseuse and is willing to give you a happy ending. (Dirty phrase: "Could you go a bit lower... lower still, yeah... that's the spot.")

6. Pretend to knock on the wrong hotel room door but the stranger who opened up (your partner) invited you in any way. (Dirty phrase: "Never mind, I could use the company of someone as gorgeous as you are right now.")

7. Play the role of a landlord who's come to collect their rent, but your partner can't pay, so they end up paying in kind. (Dirty phrase: "I'm gonna fuck my money's worth out of you tonight.")

8. Play the role of a yoga instructor teaching your partner how to stretch and bend over. (Dirty phrase: "Nice and slow... that's it. Now bring that sexy ass of yours over here.")

9. Play the role of a boss who is about to have sex with his or her employee on the desk. (Dirty phrase: "I see you've been striping me naked with your eyes all day. It's time to turn this office into our sex haven!")

10. Both of you should assume the role of angry partners in a rough sex session.

11. Play the role of a tour guide with a strong accent. Let your

partner listen to your dirty talk with a different accent.

12. Recreate the roles of your favorite porn stars from a porn scene or novel.

13. Play the role of a naughty maid trying to have quick sex with the house owner before the wife shows up. (Dirty phrase: “I’ll be in the kitchen… I’ve got no pants on. Hurry!”)

14. Pretend to be a dance teacher and seduce your student (partner) through your movements. (Dirty phrase: “Place one foot ahead of the other and move your hips this way. Gosh! You look so sexy in that pose!”)

15. Play the role of a hooker trying to get a one-night stand. (Dirty phrase: “I’m free for the whole night. Would you like to do something fun and sexy?”)

16. Play the role of a pizza guy who gets a blow job in place of cash. (Dirty phrase: “I’m sorry I don’t have any cash at home. But I’m sure we can figure out some other more interesting way to pay?”)

17. Pretend is your first sex as husband and wife on your wedding night. (Dirty phrase: “I’ve been waiting for this moment all my life. I can’t wait to finally be inside you / have you inside me!”)

18. Play the role of an artist and paint your nude partner on a canvas. (Dirty phrase: "You have the curves of a god/goddess.")

19. Play the role of a shy virgin having sex for the very first time. (Dirty phrase: "Promise to be gentle with me tonight, would you?")

20. Play the role of an innocent person who is completely naïve about sex. Let your partner teach show you how to have sex. (Dirty phrase: "Is that what an erect penis/aroused vagina looks like? Oh... I see.")

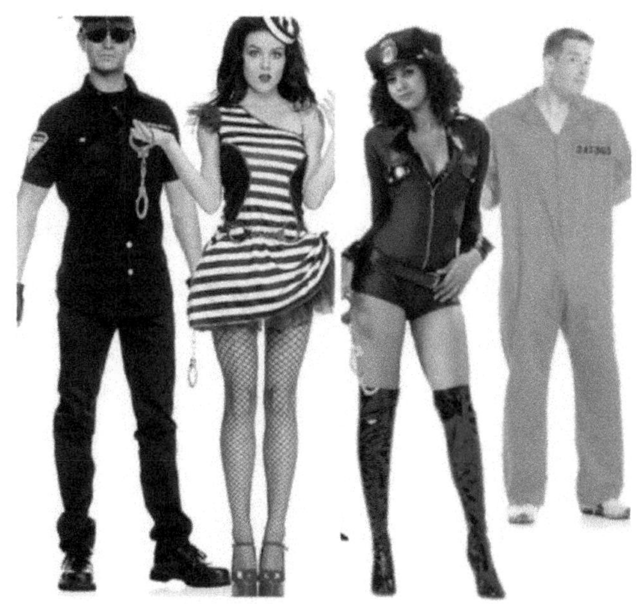

21. Pretend you are a student who's trying to seduce their teacher for better grades. (Dirty phrase: "I might not be good

at algebra, but I can tell from the way you look at me that you want to have a taste of me, don't you?")

22. Pretend that you are a hypnotist who has hypnotized your partner. Command them to do whatever you wish. (Dirty phrase: "You will suck my cock / eat my pussy when I instruct you. Nod if you understand me.")

23. Play the role of a nurse and bathe your "sick" patient (your partner). (Dirty phrase: "If you would step out of your robe. Good boy/girl. Now relax let me take good care of you.")

24. Pretend that you are a striptease and give your partner a lap dance. (Dirty phrase: "Do you like it when I bend over and shake my ass like this?")

25. Play the role of a cab driver and have sex with your client in the back of your car. (Dirty phrase: "Your destination is still a bit far. I suggest we stop here for a while, grab a quick bite and have a quickie.")

Conclusion

Tips and Tricks For The Future

As you go on in your sexual life, stay open-minded, and never stop listening to your body. People change and you will likely change as well. By being open to these changes and being receptive to them in yourself and your long-term partner, you will be able to ensure you are always getting the most out of sex. Don't forget to communicate with your partners in order to better understand them and sex in general, as communication leads to learning and this is a great thing when it comes to sex.

The hope is that this book has given you the tools you need to keep your sex life fresh and ever-changing by introducing you to the world of Kama Sutra. Maybe you have tried some of the positions from the Kama Sutra before, and you needed help in order to learn more. Maybe you are new to sex and you wanted to study up on different positions to try for beginners. You now have a whole arsenal of positions to try. Maybe you have tried all of the classics and are looking to get into something completely new and adventurous. Whatever experience you came with, I hope that you are leaving this book having learned a few new things to take with you into your sexual adventures from here forward. I hope this serves as a tool for you to explore and discover yourself and your future partners.

There is something for everyone in this book, so continue to pass it on to your friends and your partners so that we can live in a world of educated and informed sexual beings. The Kama Sutra is a guide book for love and everything involved in loving another person. It is more than just a book of sex positions, but these days most people only know it for its complex and flexibility-requiring positions for intercourse. The book of Kama Sutra includes a general guide to living well in ways other than through sex. It includes a guide to foreplay, a guide to kissing and touching, as well as other ways to achieve intimacy with your partner, such as bathing together and giving each other massages. I hope that after reading this book, you understand and can appreciate this text in a new way.

In addition to the positions enclosed in these pages, I hope that you learned how to focus on your pleasure and the pleasure of your partner, how to be present during sex, and how to become more sexually intuitive in order to feel the most pleasure possible. What a waste of pleasure it would be to always have sex in the same positions over and over and never fully reach your potential for orgasm! If you haven't already, try some of the things you've learned through reading this book, and I assure you that your sex life will be much better for it!

You are now ready to go off into the world of sexual exploration and have great orgasms from here on out. Stay curious and keep learning!